I0222609

HIIT

Beginner's Guide to Hiit & Rapid Weight Loss

(How to Achieve the Body of Your Dreams With High Intensity)

Charles Harris

Published by Harry Barnes

Charles Harris

All Rights Reserved

HIIT: Beginner's Guide to Hiit & Rapid Weight Loss (How to Achieve the Body of Your Dreams With High Intensity)

ISBN 978-1-77485-119-7

All rights reserved. No part of this guide may be reproduced in any form without permission in writing from the publisher except in the case of brief quotations embodied in critical articles or reviews.

Legal & Disclaimer

The information contained in this book is not designed to replace or take the place of any form of medicine or professional medical advice. The information in this book has been provided for educational and entertainment purposes only.

The information contained in this book has been compiled from sources deemed reliable, and it is accurate to the best of the Author's knowledge; however, the Author cannot guarantee its accuracy and validity and cannot be held liable for any errors or omissions. Changes are periodically made to this book. You must consult your doctor or get professional medical advice before using any of the suggested remedies, techniques, or information in this book.

Upon using the information contained in this book, you agree to hold harmless the Author from and against any damages, costs, and expenses, including any legal fees potentially resulting from the application of any of the information provided by this guide. This disclaimer applies to any damages or injury caused by the use and application, whether directly or indirectly, of any advice or information presented, whether for breach of contract, tort, negligence, personal injury, criminal intent, or under any other cause of action.

You agree to accept all risks of using the information presented inside this book. You need to consult a professional medical practitioner in order to ensure you are both able and healthy enough to participate in this program.

Table of Contents

Introduction

This book contains information about the new trend, High Intensity Interval Training (HIIT). In this book you will find how to start HIIT suggestions, what types of foods to eat and HIIT benefits to name a few. Towards the end of the book, numerous sample HIIT workouts are added for all training levels. These include routines that can be done at the gym, outdoors, or at home. The best part about HIIT is that it is doable and cheap; no gym equipment is required. The training will depend on your environment and what is convenient for you.

This book also tackles the benefits of HIIT training. Many studies and books have explained what HIIT can do for the body, but this book explains it clearly even to those who aren't health buffs so they could understand the message being conveyed.

HIIT is not a new type of training but has simply gone under the radar. Research continues to show its effectiveness for the cardiovascular system, fat loss, and muscle retention. One of the best examples of HIIT is the impressive physique of an Olympic sprinter compared to a long distance runner.

Lastly, I hope this book benefits you regardless of whether you are just curious about HIIT, you are an athlete seeking to increase your performance, or you simply want to lose body fat in a short period of time. This book has plenty of information and exercises that will surely help you attain all your fitness goals.

Chapter 1: What Is Hiit?

HIIT stands for High-Intensity Interval Training. This kind of training alternates between high-intensity and lower intensity workouts. It repeats this cycle for a specified period.

The HIIT originated as a training routine among track athletes. Coaches made their sprinters run at peak intensity for a period and then instructed them to run at a slower pace. They would repeat this alternating pattern for the duration of HIIT session.

When you do a high-intensity interval training session, your body is producing explosive force for a short period. This has different effects on your body depending on the type of workout you are doing.

If you are running, sprinting causes your heart rate to increase to its maximum capacity. It also causes you to use your fast-twitch muscles together with your regular muscles. These muscles are responsible for the explosive force created by sprinting. They are also more developed among sprinters compared to long distance runners. As you switch to a jogging pace, your heart rate decreases but it does not allow it to go down to your resting heart rate. You also lessen the activity of your fast twitch muscles, giving it time to recover. Training this way keeps your heart rate at a faster than normal pace for the period of your workout, increasing its efficiency.

You can also use high-intensity interval training in common calisthenics exercises. In a circuit for example, you may do high intensity moves like burpees and then switch to slower workouts like slow lunges. When you are doing burpees, your focus is on finishing the set as fast as possible. When you switch to the lunges, speed is no longer your goal. You switch your focus on keeping the correct form as you do them. You can follow the lunges with another high-intensity workout like one minute of using the jump rope.

What are the Benefits of using HIIT?

HIIT improves skills that require explosive power

High-intensity interval training came from the world of sports. Before it became a popular workout system, coaches used it to condition the body of their athletes. More specifically, coaches used high-intensity interval training to train speed runners. Sprinters differ from long distance runners because they do not need to sustain their run for long periods.

Instead, they only need a short burst of energy to win. High-intensity interval training is the perfect training regimen for types of sports that require short bursts of power and speed.

Boxers for example use this method of training when practicing their flurry of punches inside the ring. A boxer needs to move around the ring for 3 minutes straight. In this period, he or she needs to throw punches, defend himself, do footwork and use head movement to avoid getting hit. Even before high-intensity interval training became popular in the fitness world, boxing coaches already used variations of it in conditioning the bodies of their boxers.

They would make the boxer throw as many combinations as he can in 30 seconds. This would simulate the amount of time he has to land a hit when he sees an opportunity in the ring. The coach would then instruct the fighter to do slower punches like jabs and do some head movement exercises. After doing that, they would go back to the high-intensity practice of throwing combinations to the bag.

Fighters would do 3-minute circuits to simulate a boxing round. The exercises conditions the fighter's body to generate shorts bursts of power in a boxing match. It perfectly simulates the way athletes use energy in a competition. Professional boxers would do 30-40 of these circuits in a workout session. They would eventually lessen the number of training rounds as the fight date comes closer.

It can also be used in training for many other types of sports and hobbies. Long distance bikes use HIIT to practice the burst of energy that they would need when sprinting to the finish line. Basketball players use HIIT routines to simulate the burst of energy they use when in a fast break. Association football players would do the same to practice their ability to run short distances in the field when making a play, gunning for a goal or defending. HIIT makes the body burn more calories

Research had shown that high-intensity interval training results in a faster metabolic rate compared to conventional cardiorespiratory workouts. The slow and steady pace of most cardio workouts only creates a slight increase in the post-workout metabolic rate. The combination of high-intensity workouts and slower workouts increases your metabolic rate even when you only do it for a short period. As a result, you burn more calories after your high-intensity interval training sessions compared to doing regular jogs or bike rides.

HIIT produces results even when done at short periods

You do not need to do long workout periods just to get results with HIIT. Because of the amount of calories that this system burns, you will be able to burn fat and sculpt your body even by doing just 15-30 minutes of high-intensity interval training every day.

If your goal is to burn fat, the fast metabolic rate this workout system produces will help you achieve that. If you want to gain muscles, you may integrate resistance training with this system to increase mass. By forcing your muscles to generate explosive force, you will create results even if you just do 30 minutes of weight training every day.

HIIT improves your muscle definition while losing weight

Most weight loss regimens cause you to lose muscle definition. Long distance running for instance, will surely result to weight loss. However, because it does not train your muscles for strength, they will shrink as you lose weight.

You can do HIIT with a many types of workouts. You can even insert some strength training exercises to your high-intensity interval training circuit to maintain your muscles mass as you are losing fat weight.

As you lose fat weight, you will see the definition of your muscles more clearly. The curves of the muscles begin to show when you are approaching 15% body fat. Because HIIT trains your muscles to do explosive movements, they will be conditioned and they will remain huge. You need to pair your HIIT protocol with a protein rich diet to make sure that you keep your muscles well nourished.

Chapter 2: Hiit Implementation

The Required HIIT Intensity

High Intensity Interval Training is called High Intensity Interval Training for a reason. Assuming that a HIIT workout is easier than a steady-state workout based on the fact that it is much shorter is a very large mistake. During the short bursts of the workout, you should be giving absolutely everything you have in the tank. Your heart rate, if measured, would be between 90-100% of its maximum. Even within the rest or "low intensity periods" between those short bursts, your heart rate should not fall below 55-60% of its maximum. This will challenge the body's anaerobic system and cause a metabolic disturbance that will have the body burning calories for up to 48 hours afterwards.

HIIT Frequency

High Intensity Interval Training is extremely taxing on the cardiovascular, muscular, and central nervous system. It's for this reason that it is recommended that AT MOST it be performed 4 days of the week. This protocol is reserved for a trainee who performs no other types of training during his or her weekly regimen. HIIT frequency should be reduced for individuals who regularly train with weights to ensure proper muscle recovery. In the case of a weight training athlete looking to reduce fat or increase cardiovascular health, I prescribe reducing HIIT sessions to three times a week, and performing steady-state on two separate days.

Modes and Getting the Most Out Of HIIT

Contrary to popular belief, HIIT doesn't have to be the traditional grueling set of sprints or bouts of speed on the elliptical machine (although it can be). Any form of exercise that incorporates periods of high intensity separated with periods of low intensity is considered HIIT. HIIT can be worked in while swimming, rowing, performing bodybuilding circuits, or if you really want to go down that route...crossfit. Weapons of choice include kettlebells, dumbbells, exercise balls, atlas stones, sledgehammers, and wheelbarrows (for distance wheeling). HIIT as stated before is an extremely simple concept. As long as you are working at the required intensity and with indomitable commitment, you are going to see results. The results you want are only limited by what you desire. Tailoring the style of HIIT (whether it is strictly cardio, bodybuilding circuit, swimming, rowing, or Crossfit) to your own personal goals is what really matters in getting the most out of your High Intensity Interval Training.

Nutrition While On HIIT

Nutrition is a branching topic, again centered around an individual's personal goals. The main purpose of HIIT for most trainees will inevitably be for fat loss. Losing fat is not a complicated process, and is often blurred in difficulty by the media and by unmotivated people who are unsuccessful in doing it. If your goal is to lose fat while utilizing HIIT, first calculate your daily weight maintenance calories. From here, it as simple as consuming 250 calories less per day. Make 50% of those calories proteins, 25% of them carbs, and 25% of them fats. That's it. HIIT will also do you the favor of burning more calories beyond the calories that you cut in that method. For pre-HIIT workout nutrition, consume a light carbohydrate and protein source about an hour before hand. A whole banana with 2 tbsp. of peanut butter should do the trick, but obviously your carbohydrate and protein sources can be swapped out for your own preferences.

Pitfalls of HIIT

Although High Intensity Interval Training is in my opinion (as well as countless others) an invaluable tool in losing fat and improving cardiovascular health, it is in all truthfulness not suited for all trainees. HIIT is fast-paced and strenuous, which leads to a higher risk of injury. Depending on body position during exercise, blood can pool in the lower extremities or dizziness can onset. In addition, attempting to push too hard as a beginner without first progressing can lead to overly excessive muscle soreness or in the worst case, rhabdomyolysis (damaged muscle fibers breaking off and entering the bloodstream, causing poisoning of the kidneys). Practice common sense and see a doctor to diagnose any possible diseases or limitations before attempting to begin any HIIT workouts or programs.

Sample HIIT Workouts

If you've been reading this short eBook and been sold on the idea of using HIIT and reaping the benefits, then you're in luck. Here is a compilation of a few of my personally chosen HIIT workout samples for you to try out for yourself. From these templates, you can even begin to design your own personally-made routines. Is that eagerness I sense?

FIVE Beginner-Level Workouts

#1: Treadmill/Elliptical Classic HIIT

(This should take roughly 10 minutes to perform. This will not include the recommended 3 minutes of light jogging to warm up beforehand, or the 3 minutes of light jogging to cool down after the workout)

Perform 20 seconds of intense speed

Perform 40 seconds of recovery jogging.

Repeat this process 10 times.

#2: Beginner-Friendly 10 Minute Bodyweight HIIT Workout

Perform each exercise at high intensity for 45 seconds followed by 15 seconds of rest. Then move onto the next exercise. Once through the circuit, rest two minutes and repeat 4 times.

Mountain Climbers

Push-Ups

Air-Squats

Crunches

Burpees (Squat Thrusts)

Plank

Jump Squats

Jumping Jacks

High Knees

Lunges

#3: Simple Outdoor Fat-Scorcher

Find a small sized hill, an area to do push-ups at the top of this hill, and a spot to perform low-intensity jumping jacks at the bottom.

Sprint as hard as possible up the hill

Upon reaching the top of the hill, perform 15 push-ups.

Jog down the hill, and perform low-intensity (meaning don't be going insanely fast) jumping jacks for 1 minute at the bottom.

Repeat this process 10 times.

#4: 20 Minute Calorie Burner

During this workout, you will perform five different movements. For 45 seconds you will attempt to perform as many reps as possible, and then rest 15 seconds before moving onto the next exercise and repeating. There will be 3 rounds of this, and 1 minute rest between each round.

Push-ups (modified if necessary) - 45 seconds

Rest - 15 seconds

Air Squats - 45 seconds

Rest - 15 seconds

Butt Kicks - 45 seconds

Rest - 15 seconds

Tricep Dips - 45 seconds

Rest - 15 seconds

Side Lunges - 45 seconds

Rest one minute and repeat the round

#5: Butt-Toner

This is one of the most simple HIIT workouts out there and will help the ladies (and who knows, maybe guys too) get the glutes and thighs that both they and the opposite sex desire. There will be a total of five rounds, with no rest between these rounds. Get to it.

10 squat jumps

30 second wall-sit

20 Forward Lunges (10 for each leg)

30 second wall-sit

Repeat

FIVE Intermediate-Level Workouts

#1: Jump Rope Oriented HIIT Workout

50 reps of Jump Roping

1o push-ups

10 Burpees

20 High Knees

50 reps of Jump Roping

10 squat jumps

10 reverse lunges (each leg)

10 burpees

50 reps of Jump Roping

20 crunches

10 flutter kicks

#2: Stadium Runner Workout

It's time to head to your local high school football stadium and hit the bleachers. For this simple yet challenging workout, you will begin by sprinting full-steam up the stairs until reaching the top. At the top of the bleachers, you will then attempt to hold a plank for the MAXIMUM amount of time possible. You will have 30 seconds to rest before jogging back down the bleachers and immediately sprinting back up to begin the next round.

Bleacher Sprint

Max-Duration Plank Hold

30 second Rest

Jog down the bleachers

Repeat.

#3: Burpee Warfare

Burpees have been a longtime conditioning favorite of American football coaches, and with good reason. The exercise entails going from a standing position, to flat on your face, to standing again, and is extremely demanding on the body's aerobic AND anaerobic fitness level. It is recommended you perform this routine on soft running track or in grass so you can stop where you are jogging to complete the burpees.

1 Minute - Perform as many burpees as possible

1 Minute : Light jog at approximately 60% of your full effort

Repeat this process 10 times

#4: Leapfrog HIIT Workout

Perform the following exercises for two rounds, with the objective of completing these two rounds in the shortest amount of time possible.

10 Squat Jumps

20 Plyo (Jumping) Push-Ups

30 Forward Lunges (15 to each leg)

40 Box Jumps

50 Jump Rope Repetitions

Repeat.

TIP: To make plyo push-ups easier, simply perform them as a regular push-up, on an incline, or on your knees. For more of a challenge, attempt to clap your hands together mid-air as your propel yourself from the ground using your chest and triceps.

#5: 7 Minutes to Rock Hard Abs

Weighted Plank - 1 Minute

Perform as many Spiderman Push-Ups as possible in 1 Minute

30 second rest

Perform as many lying V-Ups as possible in 1 Minute

Perform as many Sit-Ups as possible in 1 Minute

30 second rest

Perform as many Seated Leg Tucks as possible in 1 Minute

Perform as many Flutter Kicks as possible in 1 Minute

FIVE Advanced-Level Workouts

#1: Bodybuilding Style HIIT: Chest and Back

Bench Press - 1o sets of 10 reps - use 50% maximum weight - 30 second rests

Dumbbell Incline Press - 3 sets of 10 reps - 45 seconds rest

Dumbbell Decline Press - 3 sets of 15 reps - 30 second rests

Cable Crossovers - 3 sets of 15 reps - 30 second rests

Wide Grip Lat Pulldown - 10 sets of 10 reps - use 50% maximum weight - 30 second rests

Barbell Bent Over Row - 3 sets of 10 reps - 45 second rests

Straight-Arm Pulldown - 3 sets of 15 reps - 30 second rests

Weighted Hyperextensions - 3 sets of 15 reps - 30 second rests

#2: HIIT Swimming "Ladder" Workout

Warm-up for 5-10 minutes with low-impact cardio exercise such as jogging.

For the following intervals, rest 10-30 seconds between swimming legs depending on your fitness level.

Freestyle stroke 150 meters at a slow pace

Freestyle stroke 120 meters at a medium pace

Freestyle stroke 100 meters at a fast (sprint) pace

Freestyle 120 meters at a medium pace

Freestyle stroke 150 meters at slow pace

Perform a light 5-10 minute cool down to conclude the workout.

#3: Pulling Power HIIT

Next to squats, the barbell deadlift is heralded as the king of all exercises. There is nothing quite as primal as ripping a heavy weight off the ground. If you're a caveman and a rock is blocking the entrance to your cave, what are you going to do? You're going to deadlift that bad boy out of the way. Combine deadlifts with HIIT and you have a recipe for bad-assery.

Perform the following circuit as many times as possible in 10 minutes.

Deadlifts - 10 reps with 65% of 1 rep-max weight

Box Jumps - 10 reps

Repeat.

#4: Boxer HIIT

Fighters are some of the most well-conditioned and shredded athletes on the planet. This workout mimics their training and will help you sculpt the physique you've been after. You will need a heavy punching bag and gloves. Aim to perform 3 rounds in the quickest amount of time possible.

20 jabs (each hand)

20 knee jabs (each knee)

40 dumbbell punches (step away from the bag and perform air-punches grasping light dumbbells. Each hand will do 20 reps)

50 reps of Jump Rope

Repeat

#5: Death Grip HIIT

Grip strength will aid in all facets of life. From carrying those 5 extra bags of groceries inside to avoid another trip, hoisting those bags of cement to the backyard to start your patio, and other...extracurricular activities...grip strength will play a large role. This workout will ramp up the fat-burning benefits due to its multiple multi-joint movements and extremely high-intensity. Are you up to it? Perform the following circuit for 5 rounds in the quickest amount of time possible.

Rowing Machine - 500 Meters at 80% effort (Alternative: 100 Yard Dumbbell Farmer's Walk - use challenging weights)

Barbell Power Cleans - 10 reps

10 Pull-Ups

Repeat.

#5: HIIT Leg Workout From Hell

Leg training has a legendary reputation for being as brutal as they come. In this case, we'll be going beyond brutal. This workout will be downright nasty, painful, and gut-wrenching. But you cannot gain without sacrifice. This workout will build large, veiny, striated quads and hamstrings while at the same time burning insane amounts of calories and fat. You will be performing two rounds, and if you've challenged yourself correctly by the end, you won't have the energy to do any more than that. Or to drag yourself back to your car. Perform the following circuit while resting only when indicated.

Barbell Back Squats - 15 reps

Leg Press - 6 reps (very heavy weight)

Rest 30 seconds

Leg Extensions - 20 reps (on last round, perform a triple-dropset upon reaching 20 reps)

Dumbbell Stiff-Legged Deadlifts - 10 reps

Rest 2 minutes

Repeat

NOTE: You may perform calf exercises of your choice following the routine if desired.

Chapter 3: Why Are Hiit Routines So Short?

When it comes to cardio, people are under the impression that longer sessions of moderate-speed cardio are the way to go when it comes to burning calories and eliminating fat. This is largely because that's the way it's been taught for decades. These people scoff at the idea of a 20- to 30-minute HIIT session because they feel 60 minutes on the treadmill at a low incline and moderate speed is the way to go.

HIIT workouts are short by design because you're expected to leave it all on the line during the high-intensity portions of intervals. Giving it all you've got during multiple intervals during a HIIT session should exhaust you to the point where you wouldn't be able to do more than a 20- to 30-minute session. HIIT should be exhausting for amateurs and veterans alike, because regardless of skill level, the exerciser is supposed to put everything he or she has into the intense intervals.

The short active recovery periods aren't anywhere near enough to fully recover. They're designed to give you a breather, so you can build up enough energy to go hard again when the next interval starts. By the time a HIIT session ends, you should be short of breath and dripping sweat, with little left in the reserves.

If you're doing HIIT right and are getting your heart rate and exhaustion level into the right zones during your intervals, you'll leave the gym feeling more tired after a HIIT session than you would if you'd done 60 minutes of steady-state cardio.

While the HIIT workout itself won't burn a ton of calories, the afterburn effect mentioned previously coupled with the calories burnt during the workout will result in more calories burnt and increased fat loss in comparison to steady-state workouts that take much longer.

HIIT routines are short because they need to be short in order to ensure the exerciser can push hard during the high-intensity intervals without having to worry about burning out before the routine is complete. They're short by design, and are highly effective because of their length.

You'll realize the same benefits and then some when comparing HIIT to longer steady-state cardio routines. It isn't the length of the workout that matters inasmuch as it's the effort put into it.

Getting Ready for HIIT

If you hop on the Internet and search for HIIT workouts with the intent of doing the first workout you find, you may be in for a rough time, especially if you've lived a rather sedentary lifestyle up until now. Even the HIIT workouts that claim to be for beginners are going to be difficult for someone who's spent a good portion of their adult life sitting behind a desk or on the couch.

That's not to say it can't be done. Where there's a will, there's a way and some people are able to push through until they get used to the harder routines.

Others will make it halfway through their first workout and call it quits, planning on trying again soon, only to wake up so sore the next morning they give up on HIIT for good. You haven't felt pain until you've pushed through a new workout that really digs into muscles you've barely moved for years. A few aches and pains that evening can turn into sharp, stabbing pains in the morning that make each and every step an agonizing ordeal.

The idea behind HIIT is to get in shape, not to needlessly torture yourself. It's best to start off slow and work your way up to the more difficult HIIT sessions. After all, what good is a HIIT session if it puts you out of commission for a week or longer because you're too sore or injured to keep working out?

The rest of the chapter discusses the preparations you should make in order to get ready to start high-intensity training. Making sure you're ready will go a long way toward ensuring you make it past the first few sessions of HIIT.

Get a Physical Exam

Before you start HIIT training, it's imperative you make sure you're physically healthy enough for such a vigorous exercise program. Vigorous exercise puts a strain on your entire body, so it's important to ensure your body will be able to handle it in advance of starting a program. The best way to do this is to visit a doctor and let him know your plans. Ask him specifically to examine you to make sure you're physically healthy enough to do HIIT.

It's a good idea to bring a notebook and a pencil to your examination. Write down the questions you plan on asking in advance of the appointment and take notes on pertinent information. It may seem like it'll be easy to remember during the examination, but you don't want to end up racking your brain for answers later on down the road if you don't take notes.

Here are some questions you should ask your doctor at the examination:

Am I physically able to perform high-intensity interval training?

This is the most important question you're going to ask, so pay close attention. Make sure your doctor knows it isn't just interval training; it's high-intensity interval training. Your doctor should be able to tell you about any health issues you have that will preclude you from this sort of training and should be able to provide guidance as to any limitations you may have. Previous or current injuries, illnesses, diseases and/or accidents may make HIIT too difficult or dangerous to perform.

Do I have any medical conditions that limit my ability to do vigorous exercise? Will I make these conditions worse by performing HIIT?

You're looking to get in shape and making current medical conditions worse is not going to help you achieve that goal. If HIIT isn't for you, your doctor should be able to help you choose a more appropriate plan or be willing to refer you to someone who can.

Are there any restrictions as to the actions I can perform? Am I taking any medications that could affect my heart rate?

Take heed of your doctor's advice when it comes to restrictions. Your doctor should be able to provide you with a list of your limitations in light of your current physical condition. Ask your doctor to provide you with a target heart rate you should reach during your workouts and for a danger zone heart rate at which you should stop working out or slow down until your heart drops to a safer level. Be aware that medications that affect your heart rate may make it difficult to use heart rate as an effective metric for measuring vigorous exercise.

Do I need to lose weight? If so, how much?

Here's another important question. Some people overestimate the amount of weight they need to lose, while others underestimate it. Your doctor should be able to give you a good idea of what a reasonable weight loss goal would be and how fast you should be trying to reach that goal.

How is my current weight affecting my health?

This question is more for motivation than anything else. If you doctor tells you you're overweight and your current weight is dangerous to your health, you should be concerned enough about your health to make the changes he or she recommends. While you're at it, ask how much weight you need to lose to improve your health. You might be surprised at how much of a difference a few pounds can make.

Learn How to Monitor Exercise Intensity

In order for HIIT to work its wonders, you have to be able to push yourself hard for short periods of time. How hard you push during these short bursts of exercise can make a big difference in the overall effectiveness of your workouts. Exercise intensity is a measurement of how hard you're working and it directly correlates to calories burned, strength gains and changes in weight, body fat and endurance.

There are a number of ways to monitor exercise intensity and some are more effective than others. When you're first starting off, even light exercise may feel intense. You aren't used to the way working out makes you feel and your body hasn't had time to adjust to your new healthy lifestyle, so you're going to feel tired rather quickly. This will change as you gain experience and your body adjusts to the exercises you're doing. Within just a few days your body will start to change.

As you gain experience and get used to HIIT, you'll need to adjust the intensity of your workouts to keep up with the gains in strength and endurance you're realizing. Don't get stuck on a certain length of time, number of exercises or amount of weight. Your HIIT routine should constantly evolve to match your current physical condition. A routine that feels mind-numbingly difficult today will be way too easy a month or two down the road.

You're going to have to constantly adjust your workouts based on your ability to push your body to its limits. In order to do that, you're going to need to know how to tell when you're nearing your limits. The rest of this section lays out methods you can use to measure exertion.

Perceived Exertion

Perceived exertion is the technical term for how tired you feel after a certain set of actions. It's measured on a sliding scale from 1 to 10, with 1 being little to no exertion being felt after completing an exercise and 10 being complete and utter exhaustion.

When it comes to HIIT, you want to push yourself to a high level of perceived exertion during the intense training sessions and then back off to a manageable level during the active recovery sessions. During the high-intensity intervals you should be reaching somewhere in the range of 8 to 10 on the perceived exertion scale. Beginners should shoot for the 5 to 7 range to start. As you improve and become an intermediate exerciser, the 8 to 9 range may be more appropriate. Elite athletes can push themselves closer to 10.

Here's a chart that shows the different levels of perceived exertion:

Exertion	Difficulty
10	Exhaustion
9	Near Exhaustion
8	Very Difficult

7	Difficult
6	Somewhat Difficult
5	Average
4	Fairly Easy
3	Easy
2	Very Easy
1	At Rest

Perceived exertion is highly subjective because some people feel fully exerted long before others will. This isn't necessarily a bad thing, because it's an individualized measurement of how tired you feel. Perceived exertion can vary from day to day and even from hour to hour dependent upon a number of external factors. It is the easiest way to measure how hard you're pushing yourself, since all it requires is being conscious of what your body is telling you—and trust when I say you'll be explicitly aware of how tired you are during a HIIT session.

You should be pushing yourself hard, but not quite to the point where you feel dizzy and are about to pass out. If you're reaching that point, you're probably taking it too far.

The Talk Test is sometimes used by those seeking to measure perceived exertion. This is a measurement of how easy it is to talk after engaging in a series of exercises. The ability to speak easily indicates low exertion, while difficulty speaking because of shortness of breath indicates higher exertion.

Target Heart Rate

Stick around the world of HIIT long enough and you'll come across literature that states you don't need to wear a heart rate monitor when you start HIIT because heart rate can't accurately be measured during a HIIT session. The reason for this is there is a lag between your heart rate and the stress your body is being placed under. It's difficult to judge exertion during short intervals by heart rate because your heart rate may not max out until you're in one of your rest periods.

This could end up being very dangerous advice.

The main reason to monitor heart rate isn't to judge when to start and stop exercises. It's to make sure your heart rate doesn't spike up to dangerous levels during the intense exercise periods associated with HIIT. Yes, heart rate does lag a bit behind, but if you hit an extremely high heart rate during exercise, you'll know it's time to back off and enter a rest period earlier than planned, since you know your heart rate might keep climbing after you enter the active recovery period.

It's understandable why some people aren't worried about heart rate during HIIT. For most healthy people, heart rate isn't going to be an issue. Your body will wear down before your heart climbs into dangerous territory and stays there.

Monitoring heart rate during HIIT is largely a precautionary tactic and it's difficult to use it as a measurement of when to start and stop intervals, but there is one good use for heart rate.

It can be useful in judging how hard you're pushing yourself. Your heart rate is a good way to measure how close you're pushing your body to its aerobic and anaerobic thresholds.

In order to use heart rate as a metric, you're going to need to know your resting heart rate (RHR), which is the number of times your heart beats per minute while your body is at rest. Generally speaking, lower numbers indicate better cardiovascular fitness. The normal range for healthy adults is between 60 and 100 beats per minute. Elite athletes can have heart rates that are closer to 40 beats per minute and some may even drop below 30, but it's extremely rare. If you aren't an elite athlete and your heart rate is consistently below 60, it's time to get in to see a doctor. You should also consult with your doctor if your heart rate is consistently above 100.

The best time to check your resting heart rate is in the morning, as soon as you wake up. Your body has been at rest all night and this is the time you're most likely to get an accurate reading. Once you've gotten out of bed and have started moving around, your heart rate will go up.

Here are three easy ways you can check your resting heart rate when you wake up in the morning:

Place your middle and index fingers onto your wrist, just below your thumb on the inside of your wrist and count the number of beats in a minute.

Place your middle and index fingers under your jawbone, at the base of where your neck and jaw meet. Slide your fingers below your jaw to the hollowed out area beside your Adam's apple. Press gently and you should feel your pulse.

Attach a heart rate monitor and record the number of beats per minute.

Of the three methods, the heart rate monitor is the most accurate, but you can get a pretty good idea of your resting heart rate using the other two.

When using your fingers to check your pulse, either count the number of beats in a full minute or count the number of times your heart beats in 15 seconds and multiply it by 4. Don't use fingers other than your middle and index finger because they can have a pulse of their own, which will throw off your count...and may scare the heck out of you. The first time I took my pulse, I recorded a whopping 120 beats per minute. I used the wrong finger and was counting double. When I checked my pulse the right way, it went down to 70 beats per minute.

For a more accurate picture of your resting heart rate, take a measurement every morning for a week. Add all of the measurements together and divide them by 7 and you'll have a clearer picture of what your average resting heart rate is.

Keep in mind there are a number of factors that can affect resting heart rate. Here are some of the factors that must be taken into consideration:

Activity level.

Body position (standing, lying, sitting, etc.).

Health issues.

Illness.

Medications.

Stress and other emotions.

Temperature.

Once you have your resting heart rate, it's time to figure out your heart rate reserve (HRR). This is the range of heart rates your body is capable of achieving. We already know your resting heart rate, so we'll set that as the low end of the reserve.

Here's an easy method you can use to estimate your maximum heart rate (MHR), which is a measurement of the highest heart rate your body is capable of. All you have to do is subtract your age from 220. Here's the formula:

MHR = 220 – (Your Age)

If your age is 36, you'd subtract 36 from 220 and end up with a maximum heart rate of 184.

While this method is quick and easy, it doesn't take non-age related factors into account. A 36-year old who is in tip-top shape could have a vastly different maximum heart rate than a 36-year old who is overweight and out of shape. To get a more accurate estimate of maximum heart rate, you can pay to take a graded exercise test, which is a test of your physical abilities. You'll be asked to perform some sort of fitness test while hooked up to any number of machines. At the end of the test, a printout will be provided that will reveal a number of metrics regarding your level of fitness. If your doctor doesn't offer graded exercise tests, ask to be referred to a clinic or medical center has them on offer.

To figure out your heart rate reserve with the information you now have on hand, subtract your resting heart rate from your maximum heart rate, as follows:

HRR = (Maximum Heart Rate) − (Resting Heart Rate)

Say the 36-year old in the previous example has a resting heart rate of 72 beats per minute and we already figured out he has a maximum heart rate of 184. We plug this information into the heart rate reserve formula, as follows:

HRR = 184 − 72

HRR = 112

This person's estimated heart rate reserve is 112. This number is useful because we can use the Karvonen formula to determine the intensity percentage of your heart rate reserve at which you should be working out.

Here is the Karvonen formula:

Training heart rate = (HRR x Intensity Percentage) + RHR

The lower boundary of the intensity percentage will be 50%. Let's plug the information we already have from the previous example into the formula:

Training HR = (HRR x 50%) + RHR

Training HR = (112 x .5) + 72

Training HR = (112 x .5) + 72

Training HR = 128

This is the lower boundary of your target heart rate percentage. 128 beats per minute is the estimated heart rate that will be reached when this person is working at 50% capacity. Training at this heart rate won't do much good.

Next, we need to figure out the training heart rate at 60%, 70%, 80% and 90%

using the same formula we just used. Here's a chart showing the training heart rates at each intensity percentage for the 36-year old we've been using as an example:

Intensity Percentage	Heart Rate
50%	128
60%	139
70%	150
80%	167
90%	173

If you don't feel like doing all of the calculations yourself, you can determine your resting heart rate and plug it into an online calculator that does all the work for you. Here are a couple sites you can use:

http://www.briancalkins.com/HeartRate.htm

http://www.sparkpeople.com/resource/calculator_target.asp

Once you have your percentages figured out, you'll have a rough idea of the heart rate zones you want to get into. Beginners will probably want to push themselves into the 50% to 70% range during intervals when first starting off. Intermediate exercisers may decide to shoot for 70% to 85% during intervals and elite athletes can push themselves to 90%. Start off slow and work your way up to the more intense intervals as you feel your body can handle them. As you gain experience, you can push yourself harder and harder until you're able to get into the higher zones.

It helps to remember that working too hard in the beginning can lead to injury and you'll burn out quickly. On the flip side of the coin, not working hard enough will result in less than stellar gains.

Keep in mind that target heart rates are estimates. Beginners may feel comfortable working at a higher intensity. If you finish a workout feeling like you didn't get anything accomplished, you may need to up the intensity the next time you do a HIIT routine. On the other hand, if you're so tired you can barely move and are still exhausted a day later, you may want to tone things down a bit. It's all about finding a happy medium and constantly adjusting your workouts in order to stay in the zone.

Check with your doctor as to the intensity percentage he or she thinks you should be reaching during HIIT. Take heed of any exercise restrictions your doctor places on you. Certain medications and medical conditions can affect your heart rate and may make it impossible to use your heart rate as a measurement of exercise intensity.

As an example, consider someone taking beta-blockers, which are a class of drugs used to reduce stress on the heart in order to treat hypertension, angina, abnormal heart rhythms or any of a number of other medical conditions. High-intensity exercise won't have the same effect on the rhythm of the heart when beta-blockers are in use, so this isn't a good measurement of exercise intensity. A person taking beta-blockers will have to use perceived exertion and/or the Talk Test in order to determine how intensely they're working out.

If you're out of shape and you find your heart rate spiking higher than it should be during or just after intervals, consult with your doctor immediately, as there may be underlying health conditions you aren't aware of that could be putting you in danger when you work out.

Set Goals

If you've made a commitment to losing weight and/or getting fit through HIIT, the best way to ensure you stay on track is to set measurable goals. Without goals, it's easy to start skipping workouts and cheating on your diet. After all, it's tough to stay focused when you aren't holding yourself accountable for your actions.

You've already got the hardest part out of the way. Most people spend more time choosing their workout plan than they do setting their weight loss goals and working toward achieving them. The fact that you've purchased this book is a big step in the right direction. Now it's time to set some realistic and measurable goals that will help further your agenda.

While researching weight loss programs and goals, you may come across a set of standard guidelines for losing weight. These may or may not be a good fit for you, based upon your current health, diet and personal ability. Your doctor and/or a personal trainer should be able to help guide you in the right direction when it comes to setting attainable goals. Don't for a second feel like you have to be shoehorned into set standards. You're an individual and your body may be wired differently than the average person the standard is designed for.

A general guideline for healthy weight loss is one to two pounds per week. Slow weight loss is believed to be better than rapid weight loss because you're more likely to be able to sustain slow weight loss over a long period of time. Rapid weight loss is usually water loss and isn't sustainable. Once the water is gone, the body will go into conservation mode and your metabolism will slow. Weight loss will stop or slow to a crawl and you'll end up frustrated and stuck at a plateau.

We've all heard the saying, "Slow and steady wins the race." This appears to hold true when it comes to weight loss and staying fit as well. What it doesn't hold true for is the high-intensity intervals you'll be doing. Those should be done as fast as you can safely do them.

In order for weight loss goals to work, they have to be measurable. Setting a goal of "I want to lose weight this year" will be significantly less effective than setting a goal that states "I want to lose 40 pounds in 12 months' time." The second goal is a specific goal that allows you to further build upon your weight loss goals by breaking them down into manageable short-term goals. In order to lose 40 pounds in a year, you have to lose just over ¾ of a pound per week. While 40 pounds may sound like a lot, ¾ of a pound per week is manageable for most people.

 Setting short-term goals allows you to adjust the intensity of your workouts and your diet if you consistently aren't reaching your short-term goals. A week or two of missed goals aren't a big deal, as long as you're making the adjustments necessary to ensure you don't consistently miss short-term goals. If you only set long-term goals and end up missing them, you could potentially end up wasting years of time instead of weeks.

This is one of the biggest pitfalls people find themselves stuck in. The new year rolls around and they declare they're going to start eating healthier, exercising and will lose the extra pounds they've packed on. They work at it for a month or two before getting side-tracked and losing interest because they either aren't seeing the results they expected or they don't feel like working out and eating right anymore. They tell themselves they've got plenty of time to reach their goal before next year gets here. Before they know it, the next year rolls around and the same thing happens. Then the next year . . . and the next year . . . and so on and so forth.

Soon, instead of a few years' worth of extra pounds packed on they've got decades worth of poor diet and lack of exercise to contend with. The body might be able to hold up under the constant bombardment of bad food and bad fitness in the short-term, but it eventually begins to fall apart.

Setting realistic goals will help you avoid the pitfall of "I'll do it this year." You're going to need to set short-term goals that you'll have to make a conscious decision to ignore. Weekly goals allow you to hold yourself accountable every single week. If you're consistently not hitting your weekly goals, you're going to be painfully aware of it.

Of course, you have to set your weight loss goals based on your current weight. If you weigh 220 pounds, then 40 pounds in a year may be reasonable. On the other hand, if you weigh 120 pounds, you're probably going to kill yourself trying to drop 40 pounds. At this point, weight loss probably isn't desirable. It would be time to start setting other fitness goals, like building endurance and improving fitness.

Once the weight loss goals have been set, try to lock in a workout schedule. While you may be tempted to workout 5 to 7 days a week, HIIT training is tough on the body and you should shoot for at least one day off between training sessions. Set an initial goal of three sessions a week and give yourself at least a day off between each session. If you want to work out more than that, you can, but be sure to choose other workout routines that don't involve HIIT.

When setting goals you also have to take any health issues you have into consideration. Diabetics and people with high blood pressure will need to set goals that are different from those who are healthy, especially when it comes to diet.

Patients with arthritis and degenerative diseases won't be able to lift as much or push as hard as those who have healthy bones and muscles.

There's a lot to take into consideration, so don't be afraid to get advice from professionals in the field of fitness and health. Your doctor may be able to help, but I'd take it a step further and also talk to a dietician and a personal trainer. They'll be able to give you more targeted advice and are more likely to be able to guide you in the right direction when it comes to setting goals.

Create a Plan

Now that you've got your goals worked out, you've got to design a plan to help you reach those goals. A goal is only as good as the plan that supports it, so this is one of the most important steps you'll take. The more planning you do, the more likely it becomes that you'll achieve your goals.

There are two plans you're going to need to create in order to ensure success:

Workout plan.

Diet plan.

We'll cover workout planning in a bit, but for now it's important to realize you should have your workouts planned well in advance. When you say you're going to work out three times a week whenever you have the time to work out, you're giving yourself an easy exit route whenever you don't feel like working out. It's all too easy to find other "urgent" issues that need to be taken care of instead of working out.

As far as diet planning goes, the best diet plans lay out meals well in advance. Creating a weekly, monthly or even yearly diet plan allows you to plan healthy meals and to purchase the items you'll need in order to make these meals in advance. Don't fall into the trap of saying, "I'm going to start eating healthy this week" without detailing exactly how you're going to eat healthy. You'll find yourself saying the same thing week after week, but taking little action in regard to actually eating healthy.

Plan every last detail, down to the snacks you're going to eat during the day. Planning three meals a day is easy, but good eating habits can seriously be hampered by a trip or two to the vending machine in the middle of day. Plan to eat healthy snacks and you'll be well-ahead of the curve when it comes to weight loss.

Don't use dining out as an excuse to eat unhealthy foods and gorge yourself. The occasional cheat meal as a reward won't do too much damage, but if you eat out all the time, you're going to need to plan your meals while dining out as well. Most restaurants have menus available online, so scope them out in advance and figure out what you're going to eat when dining out.

The crux of your diet plan should be the meals you're eating at home. Breakfast, lunch and dinner should all consist of whole, healthy foods that will make you healthier, as opposed to hampering your fitness efforts. Figure out what you're going to eat for each meal during the week and write it down.

Pick one day during the week as your shopping day and create a list of all the foods you're going to need based on your meal plan. The less time you spend at the grocery store, the better. Once you start eating healthy, you'll be amazed at the row after row of unhealthy food you now have to traverse to get to the good stuff. There's temptation around every corner (and on most of the end displays), so get in, get what you need for the week and get out, hopefully without having tossed anything unhealthy in the cart.

One trick you can use at most grocery stores is to stick to the perimeter of the store. This is where most of the healthy foods will be. You'll still have to ignore some unhealthy foods, but the middle aisles are usually packed full of processed and unhealthy foods.

While a full-scale diet plan is beyond the scope of this book, there is a ton of resources out there, both paid and free diet plans being a Google search away.

Create a diet plan and stick to it and you'll be well on your way to reaching your weight loss goals. HIIT will be the icing on the cake that tones your body and kicks your weight loss effort into high gear.

Chapter 4: Understanding The Energy Pathways

HIIT is exercise. It is movement. And even when making it fun, HIIT still entails exertion—not necessarily full, 100%, supramaximal exertion, but exertion nonetheless. That means the body is going to be using energy to fuel that exertion. And as the body uses energy, it also fatigues. To understand what is happening in your or your clients' bodies, to understand why and how the muscles fatigue (with the aim of delaying it), and to be able to design the most appropriate HIIT protocols for you or your clients, depending on starting levels of fitness, we must take a trip inside the human body. In this lesson we begin exploring the body's different paths for accessing energy.

Several subsequent lessons will explore in more depth the energy pathways from this lesson and also explain their connection to HIIT.

In order to understand the body's energy pathways, we have to start with the molecule adenosine triphosphate (ATP). ATP is the energy supplier that must be available for any muscle to move, contract, or exert force. So whether a person is petting their dog, sprinting to catch a bus, sleeping, or engaging in a HIIT workout, it is ATP that is responsible for the muscle movement. The way it works is that the ATP molecule combines with water and then splits apart to form energy—resulting in muscle contraction and a by-product molecule called adenosine diphosphate (ADP). In order for the muscle activity to continue, the limited supplies of ATP must be replenished. And that's where the various energy pathways come into play—the body has a few different pathways for replenishing that ATP—and, as you'll see, the particular pathway depends on the type of activity and the duration of the activity that the person is doing.

ATP-PC System

For high-power, short-duration activities— we're talking explosive, 1- or 2-time movements lasting a total of 10 seconds, muscles depend on the ATP-PC system. This system does not use oxygen, so it is anaerobic. What happens is the ATP molecule is broken down by the enzyme creatine kinase to become adenosine diphosphate (ADP). As I already stated, this system only allows a supply of ATP for 10 seconds, depending on how much phosphocreatine a person has already stored. If activity continues beyond this 10-second period, the body must rely on another energy system to produce ATP—the glycolytic system.

Examples of actions that engage the ATP-PC system—maximal effort sprinting, jumping, and heavy weightlifting (below 5 repetitions).

Glycolytic System

When the ATP-PC system has done its job, but the body is still demanding energy (or ATP), the next system to provide the supply is the glycolytic system. For moderate-power, moderate-duration activities—we're talking exertion that continues for 90 to 120 seconds, the body engages the glycolytic system, a process called glycolysis, for its ATP supply.

Similarly to ATP-PC system, glycolysis also does not depend on oxygen, so it too is anaerobic. For the creation of ATP, glycolysis starts with an irreversible reaction. One molecule of glucose is converted into glucose 6-phosphate by the enzyme hexokinase. In the final step of this 10-step process, phosphofructokinase (PFK-1) converts fructose 6-phosphate into fructose 1,6-bisphosphate. This last step is very important because that is when two molecules of ATP are created. In addition to ATP, pyruvate is also a product of glycolysis.

Examples of activities that engage the glycolytic system—400–1,500-meter running and hypertrophy workouts.

Oxidative System: The TCA Cycle

When oxygen is available, those pyruvate molecules created at the end of glycolysis are broken down into acetyl-CoA, which then can enter the mitochondria, into the TCA cycle, and finally through the electron transport chain to generate ATP.

The TCA cycle (Krebs or the citric acid cycle) is the body's cycle for generating energy during aerobic respiration. For activities like running a marathon, playing video games, and sleeping, the muscles in the body are receiving ATP via the TCA cycle.

The TCA cycle, consisting of 8 steps catalyzed by 8 different enzymes, takes place in the mitochondria. The pyruvate from the glycolytic pathway is converted into acetyl-CoA by pyruvate dehydrogenase.

The cycle is initiated when acetyl-CoA reacts with oxaloacetate to form citrate by the enzyme citrate synthase. In the last step of the cycle malate will be converted back into oxaloacetate by malate dehydrogenase, and now the cycle can repeat itself. This reaction will create one molecule of NADH.

The NADH and FADH2 molecules created by the TCA cycle will enter oxidative phosphorylation or the electron transport chain (ETC) where they will be converted into ATP. This process happens in the inner mitochondrial membrane.

The electron transport chain (ETC), the final step in cellular respiration, only occurs when oxygen is available. The ETC, located on the inner mitochondrial membrane, is where most of the ATP is created. Thirty-four ATP are produced from one molecule of glucose.

Examples of activities that engage the oxidative system and TCA cycle—reading, talking on the phone, walking, listening to music, and running a 10-K race.

The Big Takeaway

ATP is the molecule muscles depend on for contraction. The body has three different pathways for supplying muscles with ATP:

•For short, high-power work, the ATP-PC system creates the needed ATP. It's anaerobic.

•For moderate duration, moderate-power work, the glycolytic system, also anaerobic, is engaged.

•For long duration, low-power work, the oxidative system (TCA cycle) is engaged. This is aerobic.

Knowing the energy pathways is very important. It will help you create a variety of fun and exciting HIIT workouts for your clients that will yield noticeable, positive health benefits for them—as opposed to a limited number of workouts that only get participants extremely exhausted, which can be very uncomfortable and not enjoyable.

Chapter 5: 8 Steps To Achieve The Body Of Your Dreams Through High Intensity Interval Training (Hiit)

There are various HIIT exercises which help you achieve your fitness goal. This may be to increase strength, lose weight, improve flexibility and also build muscles. All these exercises will help you get the body of your dreams as long as you don't fall out of plan.

Before beginning any HIIT program one should allow the following questions to be their guide so as to ensure health safety:

• Do you lose your balance from dizziness?

• In the present time have you had any chest pain when doing any physical activity?

• Has your doctor ever diagnosed you with a heart condition?

• Are you under any prescription for blood pressure or heart condition?

• Do you have any bone or joint problem that can worsen if there is any change in your physical activity?

• Are you aware of any reason that you shouldn't participate in physical activities?

If your answer is yes to one or more of the questions or you are over 40 years of age and have recently been inactive you should consult a physician first before i9ncreasing your physical activity.

Health Precautions for HIIT Exercises

(a.) Before you begin HIIT exercises consult a physician first for you to ensure that your body allows the exercises.

(b.) Always begin with the easy to handle exercises before progressing to the hard ones.

(c.) Ensure you do the exercises in the frequency given and avoid overworking your body which will cause injuries.

(d.) Ensure that your HIIT exercises are done and are in line with your feeding. Always eat well as the exercises require a lot of energy.

(e.) Set realistic exercise goals that you can handle.

(f.) Be careful when you are weight training by ensuring you can lift the weights easily.

(g.) Hydrate properly as proper hydration is important to help you exercise safely.

(h.) Always stretch before and after exercise activities. If you don't stretch it increases the risk of injury.

(i.) Always wear appropriate exercise safety gear.

These HIIT exercises are a build up to 8 steps that will help you achieve your desired body size and shape.

Step 1: Tabata Method

This exercise was a discovery of scientists Dr. Izum Tabata and his team thus the name Tabata training. They proved that HIIT is more effective on both the aerobic and anaerobic systems.

Procedure

• Warm up for 3-5 minutes by doing moves like marches, stationary squats and arm circles. These aim at preparing your body for the high intensity work out and to keep you on track.

• Pick either an aerobic or anaerobic exercise that you would wish to perform e.g. pushups squats.

• Perform 20 seconds of the exercise you have chosen by inputting all efforts and energy that your body can hold.

• Rest for 10 seconds or do a less intensive exercise e.g. jogging.

• Repeat this 7 more times to make it a total of 8 sets.

• The total HIIT workout time should be 4 minutes and this exercise should be done 2-4 times per week.

• This exercise requires you to work out to a maximum when doing the high intensity exercise and also embrace the rest period. After you are through you can do stretches. It is very essential to those who are short of time and are in good shape.

Step 2: Gibala Method

It was a development of Martin Gibala. It is a very demanding form of HIIT exercise but one can work a way through it to make it easy to be done. It is short and not boring. It involves 3 minutes of warm up, a minute of intense exercise and is followed by 75 seconds of rest and finishes with 3 minutes of cooling down. It acts on burning calories, enhancing cardiovascular capacity and also one's athletic performance.

Procedure

• One should warm up for 3 minutes first.

• Pick an aerobic exercise e.g. stationary biking, stair running.

• Work intensely for 50 seconds with the chosen aerobic exercise.

• Rest for 60-75 seconds or do low intensity exercise e.g. walking, slow cycling.

• Repeat this for 8-12 sets.

• You then cool down for 3 minutes.

• The exercise should be done 3 times per week.

Step 3: Timmons Method

Was a discovery of Jamie Timmons. It entails a few short bursts of flat out intensity and is highly beneficial to one's health e.g. improves insulin sensitivity. The Timmons method compounds 3 repetitions of 20 seconds of intense cycling followed by 2 minutes of slow pedaling. It is a good method as it is effective and enjoyable.

Procedure

• One warms up for about 3 minutes.

• Pick an aerobic exercise e.g. biking.

• Do the chosen exercise for 2 minutes.

• After this relax for 20 seconds.

• Repeat 3times ensuring you do a total of 4 sets.

• You can then cool down for 3 minutes.

Step 4: Turbulence Method

It is the most efficient work out for fat loss. It was a development by Craig Ballantyne. Turbulence training entails 8 reps of weight training alternated by 1-2 minutes of high intensity cardio for 45 minute maximum. It combines weight training and cardio and is also known as circuit training.

Procedure

• This exercise should be done using heavy weight, low reps and intense cardio.

• It should take a maximum of 45 minutes and be done 3 times per a week.

• One should start with a 5 minutes warm up.

• It should be followed by 8 rep weight training sets and alternate with 1-2 minutes cardio set.

• It is recommended for people who aim at toning up, building strength and still want to lose fat and they have the time.

Step 5: Power Intervals Method

Procedure

• It is a 90 seconds work out alternated with 30 seconds rest.

• It is used for cardio activities e.g. running, rowing, swimming etc.

• One should use maximum efforts in the work set and then for the rest set use 50%.

Step 6: Stop And Go Method

Procedure

• Get on a treadmill and perform a warm up by doing light jogging for 3-5 minutes.

• Then increase the incline to about 1.5.

• Get to the side of the treadmill and set the intensity to a point that you will be doing an ALL OUT SPRINT.

• Get back onto the belt and sprint for 15 seconds and you should hold the railings as the treadmill will still be moving.

• Jump back to the sides still holding the railings and rest for 10 seconds.

• Repeat steps 4 and 5 for 10-12 minutes.

Step 7: Peter Coe Method

It is a type of HIIT training with short recovery periods. It was a discovery of an athletics couch Peter Coe. The method includes sessions repeating cycles of a 200m sprint with 30 seconds rest in between.

Procedure

• Warm up.

• 200m intense running.

• 30 seconds of recovery between each fast run.

Step 8: Billats 30-30 Regime Method

It is a workout coined by Veronique Billat. The workout was aimed at allowing runners to spend the greatest amount of time at VO2 max.

Procedure

• 10 minute warm up of easy jogging.

• Run 30 seconds at your VO2 max.

• Jog 30 seconds of half VO2 max.

• Repeat the process until you can no longer cover the distance at VO2 max and this should be around 16-24 intervals.

• Cool down 10 minutes with easy jogging.

Tips For Proper HIIT Training

(a.) Make HIIT more intense for you to achieve maximum results.

(b.) Timing is of essence.

(c.) Pick a method and always complete your workout.

(d.) Focus on your breathing.

(e.) If you are a beginner start with the easy workouts as you progress.

Chapter 6: Hiit Vs Liss – Which Is Best For Weight Loss?

HIIT – High Intensity Interval Training

LISS – Low Intensity Steady State

How many times have you gotten half way through a long exercise routine and truly wondered if it is doing you any good? Is this really the way to go to get to your end goal? It really doesn't matter what that goal is whether it is to run further or faster, to sleep better, to burn more fat or be able to exercise for longer, it is very important that you realize that not all types of cardio are the same.

This is more so for when you go running but there are two cardio exercise types to consider – HIIT and LISS. So, what are the differences between these two types of cardio exercise and how do they affect your goals? More importantly, how do they affect how quickly you can reach your goals?

Cardiovascular Exercise - LISS vs HIIT

Cardio exercise is any type of exercise that raises your heart rate. All cardio exercise is designed to give your heart a workout and your circulatory system, increasing the flow of blood through your body, basically to keep you moving. However, not many people realize that the human body has three energy systems and it is important that you understand these to understand the differences between LISS and HIIT:

The Phosphagen System

The phosphagen system is the energy system that is kick-started in the initial 10 seconds of any movement. It is used mainly when you do short intense bursts of exercise. The human body stores ATP, phosphates and creatine and it calls on these stores to generate that energy within the first 10 seconds. The phosphagen system is very helpful for anyone who wants to improve performance during explosive or rapid movement.

Although this includes HIIT, most people who exercise, typically runners though, do not see the Phosphagen system as important as finding out about the differences between the other energy systems. All you need to know is that this is the system that comes into play when you begin to move.

The Anaerobic System

This is the system that gets used as energy for intensive exercise bursts of 10 seconds to 2 minutes. The anaerobic system is the one that is most utilized during a proper HIIT workout and during this short time period, glycogen stores from the muscles is used – as of yet, no oxygen has been used in the process of energy transfer.

Doing HIIT and anaerobic training a couple of times a week is a fantastic way to building up strength and speed, increasing your endurance levels, burning off more calories, even while you are sleeping, boosting metabolism and improving your performance overall. It also helps to boost cardiovascular benefits, burn more fat and preserve your lean muscle mass.

However, anaerobic training is very intense and shouldn't be done on a daily basis – your body needs decent recovery and healing time so only do it one or two times a week. HIIT pushes your body's threshold in terms of anaerobic to carry on doing high intensity exercise so the body will experience something called after burn. This is where it can take your body several hours to return to a homeostatic state – basically, your energy-in, energy-out needs to be rebalanced. However, although you should not be doing HIIT every day, you will still burn off calories even when you have finished the workout so calorie burning can even take place while you are sleeping.

The talk test is the best way to test if your training is anaerobic – you shouldn't be able to speak one word, let alone hold a normal conversation during anaerobic exercise. Do push yourself as far as your physical limits will allow but keep your form. If your form fails, you need to stop.

The Aerobic System

Once the two minutes is up, your body will begin using oxygen for its energy in the muscular system. Aerobics can be for 10 minutes up to as much as two hours because the oxygenated blood is taking energy to the muscles that you are using.

If you were a runner then long-distance running or training for a marathon would be the best examples of aerobic training and LISS, being low intensity and long in duration, is a good example of that type of training. LISS is best for increasing energy, strengthening the heart, getting the blood flowing better, good cardiovascular health and fat burning, although the fat burning only really happens in the initial workout stages.

However, the adaptation principle comes into play here and the body will adapt very quickly to becoming more efficient aerobically. This means that, if you only do

LISS and never do HIIT, it will end up being counter-productive to what you are trying to achieve, especially for maintenance and fat burning are your goals.

Because this adaptation is very quick, to keep up with it and maintain your calorie burning levels, you would need to run longer and further each time and that is why you should balance LISS and HIIT to get the best results – your body has to keep on guessing and you won't get to a cardio plateau.

You should aim for a certain amount of LISS in your daily regimes if only because of the huge benefits it brings in terms of cardiovascular health. But, if your goal is to be stronger, faster, and fitter, and have better endurance, as well as making the most of a much faster and more efficient metabolism, you should do HIIT workouts one or two times a week as well.

With any luck, the comparison between the energy systems in the human body has shown you how best to use LISS and HIIT more effectively to attain your goals. You should also now have a much better understanding of what is going on in your body when you do cardiovascular exercise. This can help you to make your routines far more efficient and speed up reaching those goals.

Chapter 7: Creating A Physical Activity Program

Following a good physical activity program can keep you in top shape. Exercising on a regular basis and just keeping yourself moving can help you avoid a variety of diseases. You will also be able to get a ripper body. Then again, how can you develop an ideal HIIT workout program?

Well, you should keep in mind several factors. It is very important for you to consider the intensity, frequency, and duration of your work intervals as well as the length of their recovery. The intensity for a high intensity work interval should range at eighty percent of your estimated maximal heart rate.

This work interval must make you feel like you are exercising very hard. You can use the talk test as a guide. If you find it difficult to carry a conversation, then this is an indication that you are doing fine. The intensity of your recovery interval should be forty to fifty percent of your estimate maximal heart rate.

Things to Keep in Mind Before Beginning the Program

If you do not want to encounter any problems, see to it that you take a fitness test. You can also increase your activity level substantially. Here are some questions that you need to answer in order to make sure that you are physically ready for your exercise program or routine.

Has your physician ever told you that you have an existing heart condition or that you need to engage in physical activity only if recommended by a medical professional?

Do you experience chest pain whenever you engage in physical activity?

Have you had chest pain when you were not participating in any physical activity for the past month?

Do you feel dizzy and then lose your balance? Do you lose consciousness?

Do you have an existing joint or bone problem that can be worsen by a change in your routine or physical activity?

Does your physician prescribe medication for your heart condition or blood pressure?

Are you aware of any reason why you must not engage in physical activity?

If you answered 'yes' to at least one of these questions, if you are worried about your health, or if you are at least forty years old and have been inactive, you should consult your doctor before you increase your level of physical activity or take a fitness test. On the other hand, if you answered 'no' to every question, then you can safely start the exercise program.

Once again, you should get medical evaluation and clearance before you begin performing HIIT exercises. Keep in mind that not all programs are ideal for everyone. Some programs may even cause you to have injuries. Your activities should be comfortable for you. In case you encounter discomfort or pain, it is advisable that you discontinue the program immediately and obtain medical consultation.

Chapter 8: Creating The Perfect Hiit Workout To Help You Lose Weight

The beauty in HIIT workout is that to work, it must be customized and personalized. HIIT will not work the same way for me, for you. Remember that high-intensity interval training aims to push the individual body to the limit. It goes without saying that each person's body is different. The high-intensity interval training that a fitness buff will engage in will not be remotely close to the one an obese person will engage in. One person may engage in a routine for 20 minutes thrice weekly and come out with more results than another person doing the same routine for the same period. This is obviously because the routine was pushing the first person's limit and was not doing the same for the second. Hence, you must know and understand how to design your own HIIT workout.

However, it does not end there. Your primary aim is to lose weight and not to gain muscle. For this reason, whatever routine to make must be aimed at losing weight. This is why you must not just engage in just any high-intensity interval workout. You must make research to see if it offers your body what it needs for losing weight. Here is the best way to design your own high-intensity interval workout.

Picking the Exercises

At this stage, you should pick out some of the cardiovascular exercises you are familiar with. Here are a few of the beneficial cardiovascular exercises for weight loss. You will ideally need a routine of about 110-15 exercises. Your exercises will fall into four groups namely cardio exercise, upper body exercise, lower body exercise, and finally core exercise.

Cardio Exercise

Burpees

Jumping Squats

Diamond Jumps

Squat Jumps

Jogging in Place

Jump Rope

Running up and downstairs

Mountain climbers

Skaters

Sit Outs

This is the first group of exercises. Pick any seven workouts that you are familiar with. Ensure that you know the proper form to take with the seven exercises you have chosen so as not to mar your progress.

Upper-Body Exercise

Bench press

Push-Ups

Shoulder press

Triceps dips

Back squat

Overhead press

This is the second group. In this group, you are to pick any 3 exercises you are familiar with. These exercises are to build your lower body. When you decide on three, ensure that you perfect the form and move to the next group to select.

Lower-Body Exercise

Dead Lifts

Donkey Kicks

Skater Lunge

Pistol Squat

Sprints

Diamond Jumps

In this third section, the exercises here are mean to develop your lower body. They are often referred to as lower-body exercises. In this section, pick three. When you have three picked out, work on your form to ensure you know how to carry out the exercise.

Core Exercise

The Plank

Reverse Crunch

The Dead Bug

V-Ups

Bicycle Crunches

This is the last section you need to pick from. The exercises here are exercises that build your core. In this section, you need to pick two exercises. Here, you pick the exercises that you are familiar with. When you have picked, you should go on to ensure that you have the right form and know exactly how to do the exercise.

Picking out your exercises is actually simple but should be done tastefully. When the exercises are picked out, you can move to the next stage.

Chapter 9: Welcome To Cycling 2.0 (Gadgets, Apps & More)

When you do venture out into the open road, you should make sure that you are ready for anything. You need be aware of your body condition at all times. You should also anticipate problems that may happen on the road and take measures to prepare for them. Here are some of the things that you will need for your cycling hobby:

Road Bike

The best type of bicycle for you is a road bike. These are built for speed and toughness. They are not as tough as mountain bikes but most of the good brands of road bikes can carry you and the equipment in your back for long distances.

Navigation gadgets

If you are travelling in an unfamiliar area, having a standalone GPS device will prevent you from getting lost. A lot of people argue that you should just bring your smart phone with you and use the built-in GPS. However, phones are pretty fragile and may break with minor bumps on the trip. It's safer to have 2 navigational gadgets with you.

Smart phone

Your smart phone will enhance your biking experience. Using free and paid apps, you will be able to track your trips, the distances you covered, and even the calories you burned. You could even share your workout stats with your friends on social media. Here are some of the apps that allow you to do all these and more:

Map My Ride GPS Cycling Riding

This app on Android allows you to record everything about your cycling performance. It allows you to navigate your route, measure your pace, use the GPS feature of your phone, measure the distance you've travelled for the day, and even present some of the data in sleek looking graphs. It is available in free and paid versions. The paid or MVP version features a real time locator that allows you friends and family to find you during your trips, a heart rate data analyzer and all the other features in the free version without the ads. They also have goal setting feature in the website that recommends are personal training plan available for paying users.

Strava Running and Cycling GPS

This app has similar features as the one above but it has the added feature of making your hobby social. Aside from being able to share your activities to your social media accounts, you will also be able to compare your performance with an online leader board. If you like competition, this is the app for you.

Size My Bike

This is a paid app that allows you to learn about the right bike size for your body dimensions. If you are planning to buy a new road bike, this app will be able to help you find the one that has the best fit for you. Finding the right bike will make your trips more comfortable.

Pro Cycling News

If you are hooked to the world of pro cycling, you should consider using this app. It's free and it aggregates the best cycling news as they are reported by online sources using RSS feeds. It also includes tweeter feeds of cycling's big names.

Basic bike repair tools

You should also have these tools with you especially when on a long distance trip:

Lights

Repair kits

Inner tube repair kit

Spare tube

Air pumps

Spare brake blocks

Spare break cables

Chain breaker

Extra spokes

Allen wrenches of various sizes

Lube

You should learn how to use these tools and spare parts by attending a bike repair class or by learning through the internet. There are a lot of Youtube videos devoted to this subject.

Safety

Safety is the number one reason for all this preparation. You will be able to prevent most of the problems by planning your trips ahead of time.

Planning

While planning a cycling trip, you need to consider the following factors:

Route

You should memorize where you are going and all the landmarks that you need to pass through. If you enjoy going fast, you should plan to go through roads that are good for sprinting. This means that you need to avoid road types that are prone to accidents.

Rest stops

You should also consider where you will take a break. You could take a break anywhere in the wilderness but it is much better if you can find some comfortable areas along your route where you can avail of some modern commodities.

Food and water

Some of the things that you need to consider are food and water. For day trips, you just need to learn what restaurants are in your route. You don't have to worry too much about gaining weight or fat if you eat too much because you will easily burn the food you eat during these trips.

Water is a bigger problem especially in long trips. Carrying too much water will increase the weight in your back significantly. To effectively manage your water intake, drink a lot of water in your planned rest stops. Never forget to fill up your containers before leaving. Try to conserve water in the early parts of the leg.

Repair shops along the way

You should also consider the possibility of your bike breaking down. There are some types of repairs that cannot be handled by your repair kit. If you are just biking around your home town, you can easily locate a good bike or welding shop to get your bicycle repaired. In long cross country trips however, you need to be able to locate the nearest repair shop.

Fortunately, we have the internet to help us out with that one. Plot out your trip in a map and mark where the nearest repair shops are. Make sure that they are open on the days that you will be in town.

Weather and wind

Just like in planning any outdoor occasion, you will need to plan for the weather. Try to avoid areas that are prone to landslides during the rainy season. You should also avoid steep downhill slopes on these days. Your clothing will also depend greatly on the weather forecast for your trip. Learn as much as you can about this factor to avoid being underdressed for the occasion.

The wind is also an important factor for cyclists. Some areas with strong gusts will sweep you off the road. Riding against the wind requires a lot more effort and it will tire you out easily. You may not be able to stick to your itinerary because of an unforeseen series of headwinds. When researching about the wind, you should consider the area's reputation and the time of the year.

First Aid Kit

You should also carry a first aid kit equipped with bandages and solutions for wounds and medications for common types of illnesses. In long trips, these medications can be life savers.

Camping equipment for long trips

If you plan to spend the night in the wilderness, you need to be prepared with the right camping equipment. The key to choosing the right equipment is portability. When choosing your tent for instance, you should make sure that it does not take up a lot of space and it is easy to carry.

Clothing and safety gear

Good quality cycling shorts

Not wearing the right clothing may result to damaged skin due to friction with the fabric. This usually happens in the groin area where the skin makes contact with the chair. To avoid these types of injuries, you should make sure that you wear certified cycling shorts with padding.

Helmet and pads

The best types of helmets for road cycling are the aerodynamic cycling helmets or aero helmets. Their shape allows the wind to pass smoothly and minimize the wind resistance. You should also use cycling clothes with built in pads to protect you from crashes.

Rain gear

You could also add a rain jacket during the rainy season. Cycling through the cold may lower your immune system. Using a cycling rain jacket will maintain a warm temperature in your torso even in the rain.

Don't leave home without the following:

Insurance

Make sure that your insurance covers cycling related accidents. Being active outdoors may be seen by some insurance companies as an added risk. Make sure that your hospitalization and life is covered by adding the necessary policy riders.

Let people at home know where you are going

Before leaving home, you should also tell the people you live with where you are going and how long you will be gone. If you can't arrive on time, you should let them know about it through a phone call or an SMS.

Chapter 10: Quick Start Guide

Intermittent fasting and high-intensity interval training improve blood glucose, increase growth hormone, and increase fat oxidation, according to several studies. [38] Other studies find that the combination improves brain function. [39]

While there are several varieties of intermittent fasting, the essential feature is the same: a brief fasting period, typically less than twenty-four hours, followed by a feeding period, usually between 4 to 8 hours.

The exercise protocol that is most accessible to those just beginning interval training is the 8:12 protocol, in which you exercise intensely for eight seconds and rest for twelve seconds before repeating the next round.

Intermittent fasting should not be done every day; two eighteen-hour fasts per week are sufficient to gain most of the health benefits of intermittent fasting.

You will benefit from high-intensity interval training with only three twenty-minute sessions each week. Anything more is likely to lead to burnout.

Combine intermittent fasting with strategic exercise, such as leisurely walks at the beginning of a fast and high-intensity interval training at the end, to optimize your results. Add interval training only after you've given your body a chance to adapt to the stresses induced by brief fasting. For most, the adaptation to short-term fasting takes about two weeks.

Fiber, healthy fats, and the branched-chain amino acids help to minimize hunger and promote the retention of lean body mass and loss of adipose tissue. For these reasons, I recommend adding them to your program.

Supplements

Branched-Chain Amino Acids (BCAAs): Five grams immediately before and after exercise sessions.

Omega 3-Fatty Acids: Two grams in the morning and two grams in the evening.

Fiber: Five grams in the morning and five grams in the evening.

Creatine (optional): Three to five grams in the morning.

Sample Schedule

Sunday

6:00 pm: Begin 18-hour fast. Take a leisurely thirty-minute walk in the early evening.

Monday

11:00-noon: High-intensity interval training: 8:12 x 60 rounds for a total of twenty minutes.

Noon-6:00 pm: Feeding period. Follow a nutritionally-balanced diet such as the Zone diet.

6:00 pm: Take a leisurely thirty-minute walk.

Tuesday

All day: Follow a nutritionally-balanced diet.

6:00 pm: Take a leisurely thirty-minute walk.

Wednesday

11:00: High-intensity interval training: 8:12 x 60 rounds for a total of twenty minutes.

Noon-6:00 pm: Follow a nutritionally-balanced diet.

6:00 pm: Take a leisurely thirty-minute walk. Begin second 18-hour fast.

Thursday

Noon: Fast ends.

All day: Follow a nutritionally-balanced diet.

6:00 pm: Take a leisurely thirty-minute walk.

Friday

11:00 am: High-intensity interval training: 8:12 x 60 rounds for a total of twenty minutes.

All day: Follow a nutritionally-balanced diet.

Saturday

All day: Follow a nutritionally-balanced diet.

Chapter 11: Losing Weight With Hiit

Choosing the HIIT approach over long cardio sessions is a more effective avenue to weight loss. With combining anaerobic activity in shorter workouts, your body will be building muscle and burning fat throughout the day.

The bottom line is that you can burn more calories with a 15 minute HIIT workout than a steady cardio workout. Studies have shown that after high-intensity training for six weeks, the participants received a number of benefits, including:

• A higher metabolic resting rate for up to 24 hours after their exercise session.

• A lower appetite.

• Higher levels of hormones that help fat loss.

• Improve sensitivity to insulin.

Most people today are short on time and energy. By working out the HIIT way you can increase your energy and reduce your workout time while increasing results.

Other Health Benefits of HIIT

Not only can you lose weight with H IIT, but research has shown that you can greatly improve your overall health and your fitness level. Here are some additional benefits:

With many traditional exercise and diet programs. It can be difficult to keep muscle mass. When you're losing fat. HIIT lets you build and maintain muscle mass while you're burning calories.

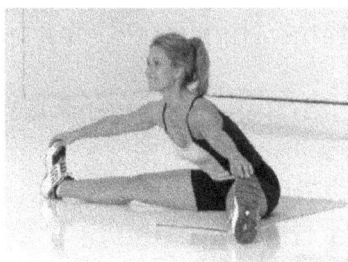

Simulates HGH production. Human growth hormone production in our body tapers off as we get older. This hormone is important for slowing the aging process, and each HIIT workout increases HGH in some cases by up to 400%, so you'll feel younger.

Improves blood sugar. Those with type II diabetes improved their blood sugar regulation after only working out two weeks with H IIT HIIT and doing three sessions weekly.

Chapter 12: Example Hiit Workouts

Here's a couple basic workouts that you can start on and how to scale them to your individual skill level:

Simple but effective

Beginner	Intermediate	Advanced
15 Second Sprint	30 Second Sprint	45 second Sprint
45 Second Rest	30 Second Rest	15 Second Rest

*Note: This chart is a very, very, generalized guideline, tailor your workout to what works best for you!

Feel free to replace "Sprints," with literally any exercise! If you're looking for the best caloric burn I suggest sticking with cardio type exercises such as:

● Sprints (see above)

● Cycling

● Swimming

● Jump Rope

● Rowing

● Stairs

Or maybe even running up and down that hill in your backyard? You really have no limits with HIIT! You can also do the same thing with the cardio exercise but pick one body weight movement and do that for your sprint intervals, but to change the difficulty we'll actually scale the movement. For example:

Body Weight Pummeler

Beginner	Intermediate	Advanced
30 Seconds Half Squats	30 Seconds Full Squat	30 seconds Jump Squats
30 Second Rest	30 Second Rest	30 Second Rest

From one exercise we literally created 3 different/unique workout by making the base exercise (squats) just a little bit harder.

We could also use the same methodology but with a push-up!

(Another) Body Weight Pummeler

Beginner	Intermediate	Advanced
30 Seconds Push-up on Wall	30 Seconds Push-up from Knees	30 seconds Full Push-up
30 Second Rest	30 Second Rest	30 Second Rest

If we wanted to make it advanced plus we could make it plyo push-ups! Feel free to change push-ups (and squats from the chart earlier) to any exercise you want! Or even use the workouts we provided. Realistically though you want your workout to be at least 5 minutes long to get some stimulus.

Some more example workouts using the methodology we taught in the earlier chapter:

(Feel free to scale them to your skill level!)

Corrrrrre!!!

30 Seconds Sit-ups

15 Seconds Rest

30 Seconds Leg Raises

15 Seconds Rest

30 Seconds Planks

15 Seconds Rest

30 seconds Russian Twist

15 Seconds Rest

30 Seconds Flutter Kicks

15 Seconds Rest

Complete as many rounds as desired

Upper Body Blaster

20 Seconds Push-ups

20 Seconds Rest

20 Seconds Plank Marches

20 Seconds Rest

20 Seconds Hands Shoulder To Overhead

20 Second Rest

Complete as many rounds as desired

Lower Body Killer

(Advanced)

45 Seconds Squat

15 Second Rest

45 Seconds Lunge

15 Seconds rest

45 seconds Calf Raises

15 Seconds Rest

45 Seconds Side lunge

15 Seconds Rest

Complete as many rounds as desired

Total Body Explosion

(Advanced)

30 Seconds Jump Squats

20 Seconds Rest

30 Seconds Plyo Push-up

2o Seconds Rest

30 Seconds Jump Lunges

20 Seconds Rest

30 Seconds Burpees

20 Seconds Rest

Considering the objective of this book is to get you programming HIIT workouts on your own we will spare farther examples.

Chapter 13: Precautions

It has proven that in a short period of time, high intensity interval training will help you boost your metabolic rate, improve your heart condition, increase insulin sensitivity, and give the best shape you desired.

But HIIT is not that easy to do. There are things to keep in mind as you work for your dream size and shape. HIIT was originally designed for experienced exercisers. If you're a beginner, you need to follow safety considerations while doing the routine.

Here are some of the safety instructions that you should always remember.

Always warm up

This is the basic safety precautions. Every exercise and game should always start by warming up. You might accidentally pull a muscle or tendon by not doing so. In addition to that, if the body is not prepared, a sudden stress on the heart with higher intensity exercises might cause some heart issues and that could be fatal. Warm up for at least 5 to 10 minutes and stay safe.

Know your intervals

Be familiar with your intervals. If you're just a beginner, don't push yourself to the limit. Use shorter intervals with longer rest periods in between. Don't ignore yourself if you really feel too much pain and tiredness. Begin with 30 second interval and 90 seconds active rest periods. Don't force it when you're just a beginner.

Have a good schedule

Intense exercise should not be done daily. Schedule your workout session wisely. Have a two to three sessions per week depending on how intense your workout is. Don't have HIIT sessions daily because you also need to have time to recover and rest.

Maintain good form

Manage to have a good shape. Be attentive to your form as the pace picks up. Be alert and cautious to avoid yourself being at risk for injury.

Monitor your intensity

The intensity should always be checked. The intensity increases as you go through different exercises. You'll be more vulnerable to injury you're your muscles are fatigued and your form gets sloppy.

That's it! By doing these safety precautions, you'll surely have successful high intensity interval training.

Chapter 14: Meditation & Visualization (In Depth)

Before you can easily combine the 2 forces of meditation & visualization you really need to have practiced both. If you've never meditated before, the benefits of meditation are that it helps you to restore energy levels & to remain focused & relaxed. Thus, you should already see that there's a link between meditation & visualization because both allow focus – one on inner harmony & the other on what it's that you really need in your entire life to make you feel good about life.

Meditation

Sit in a comfortable position. There's no need for clever crossing of legs for this kind of meditation. You must be comfortable. If you look at the position of this lady's head, it is really perfect for breathing in fresh air. If this means being seated on your favorite beach or next to your pool, then that's such a good place, but you can also do this indoors. Make sure that your clothing isn't restrictive & that you feel totally comfortable before you just start to do the breathing exercises.

You'll be just breathing in through the nose, holding the breath inside your abdomen & then simply breathing out from the diaphragm for a slightly longer count than your exhale.

Think of it in this way:

1. Breathe in, sensing the air entering your body & concentrating totally on it – Count 8

2. Retain the air – Count 6

3. Breathe out from the diaphragm – Count 10

Do this over & over, breathing in through the nostrils & out through the mouth being totally aware of the passage of air through your whole body. Take your mind off anything that actually disturbs you. Your only thought during this process should be your breathing.

Once you've achieved the ability to just concentrate solely on your breathing, do this for a period of about 10 minutes. This sharpens up your whole mind & allows it to focus well. The oxygen pumping through your system will actually help to calm you.

Visualization

Retain the same stance, though this time, when you just breathe in, think in your mind of what it's that you want to visualize. This could be such a peaceful emotion. It could be the feeling of financial reward or success, or it could be really anything that your heart does desire.

As you breathe inwards, speak words that reinforce what it's that you visualize. For instance:

"I really feel great energy."

"I feel great wealth."

And as you exhale, you really feel all that energy flowing from your body to the outside world, to be brought back in again on the next breath.

Keeping visualizing in this manner & remember that your visualization has to become such a part of your everyday life or the desired outcomes won't happen. It may've taken me half a century to just get to play the piano to any concert standard, but I did it by reinforcing the idea regularly. What I could've done is let the worldly affairs that were happening in my life simply take precedence & forget the dream. Had I done that, I may never have simply learned to play the piano. However, my dream or visualization was so strong that it actually became part of who I was, & so should your wishes.

You've to just incorporate both meditation & visualization into your life for your visualizations to bear fruit & come true. Do not wish for the physically impossible to achieve because it won't happen. If you've straight hair & want it to curl, you'll have to curl it. It isn't about what you look

156

like. It is about how you feel & what you achieve in life. If you really want to just feel more beautiful than you do, then of course, visualizing yourself as a beauty will actually help you to generate the kind of aura that goes with beauty.

Look closely at someone you simply notice as being beautiful. When you first look, your impression is that the person has great beauty. What that person probably has is really great presence & that's a totally different thing. It does not matter that her nose may be crooked or her eyes a little smaller than she'd like. She gives the impression of beauty because it is what she feels inside herself. Thus, anyone can achieve that feeling & is really able to project it to others by believing themselves to just be what it's that they seek to be.

Chapter 15: Guidelines For Hiit Workouts

* Always warm up for about 8-15 minutes with "sub-intervals" that start out lightly and gradually escalate in intensify. If you're in poor physical condition, take 20 minutes before you get to your first true work interval. HIIT on hard surfaces involving running sprints, or hard runs up hills or treadmill inclines, should get a longer warm-up for any level of fitness when compared to HIIT on a pedalling machine, due to less impact.

* Always cool down for 10 minutes.

* Keep hydrated.

* Don't overdo it or rush into things. If you're out of shape, you must build up to

faster or harder work intervals. You may need to quit the session prematurely due to burning calves, for instance, even though you still have plenty of energy.

* Make sure you wear top quality athletic shoes.

* When doing HIIT on the elliptical, stair machines and treadmill, do not hold onto the machine except when you're changing the settings or drinking water. More on this later.

* Do not assume you're not fit enough to do HIIT. Being fit is not a requirement; it's a result. The only thing that a high level of pre-existing fitness influences is mode of workout and features like speed or jumping height. Even if you're a 300 pound smoker, you'll be able to do some degree of HIIT (or at least sub-HIIT to start), even if it's just light trotting in place. If you're

concerned about your health, heart and/or weight, consult with your doctor for a complete physical prior to embarking on HIIT.

Use the RPE: Rating of Perceived Exertion

The RPE will help you determine if you're going at or very near to all-out effort, versus performing at only a moderate level (which isn't sufficient enough to unleash the metabolic cascade I described earlier).

The RPE is a scale from 1 to 10. One is how you'd feel if you were relaxing in a hammock on a breezy Saturday afternoon, sipping lemonade. Ten is how you'd feel if you were trying to outrun a charging bear—up a hill. Sometimes, the analogy is that of trying to outrun a freight train. But you get the picture.

So 5 would be moderate level effort. Seven would be challenging. Eight would be difficult. Nine would be pretty nasty. Nine and a half would be wicked. Ten would be agony.

When performing HIIT, regardless of the mode (running, walking, incline dashing, kicking a heavy-bag, pedalling a bike, stepping on a platform), you should aim for a 9 or 9 and a half for the work interval—at a minimum. Shoot for a 10 if you're up to it.

For the aforementioned "sub-HIIT" style, this would be a 7 and a half to 8 and a half. Drop below 7, and you won't be able to create that fat burning hormonal environment that's initiated with the lactate.

Use Breathlessness to Gauge Intensity

In addition to the RPE, you can do the talk test. If you can talk at the end of a work interval, it isn't intense enough. I don't mean blurt a word or two, but complete a sentence. You should not be able to speak a sentence without difficulty. You should be gasping, heavily panting, breathless but not feeling like you're going to pass out.

Ever see marathon runners cross the finish line? Do they look breathless? Often, they'll continue running, waving at the crowd. This is a stark contrast to what a sprinter does after crossing the finish line.

The sprinter will decelerate and then come to a dead stop, hands on palms, heaving for air. Or, they'll walk around after decelerating, gulping air, unable to speak. This is how you should feel at the end of your work intervals.

But remember, it's not about speed. It's about effort. That world-class sprinter feels just as pummelled at the end of the race as does a 300 pound smoker who just walked 3 mph on a 15 percent incline for 20 seconds. It's all relative!

Use Time to Gauge Intensity

Some HIIT schemes are based on a work interval of 30 seconds. Thirty seconds is about the limit before the degree of metabolic cascade loses its maximum punch. It's still there beyond 30 seconds, but for maximal results, your all-out effort needs to end in under 30 seconds.

If after 30 seconds, you stop, but you feel you could have gone for 32 seconds, you weren't moving hard enough. Thus, you must make an adjustment. It's better to wipe out after 25 seconds than to feel you could have stretched it beyond 30 seconds.

Common Mistakes

Perhaps the biggest mistake is that of overestimating effort level. This means that you've rated yourself an RPE of 10 when it's actually a 6 or 7. When a person makes this error, they automatically stop after 30 seconds or less, because that's what the instructions are, rather than being forced to stop due to complete depletion of energy.

Other mistakes:

* Improper warm-up. This can lead to strained or pulled muscles, or a feeling of being overwhelmed.

* Lack of hydration. This can lead to cramping in the abdominal area or even in a leg.

* Believing that the difficulty of the workout is related to failure or a hopeless level of conditioning, instead of

recognizing it for what it is: high intensity interval training! It's supposed to be nasty!

* Fixating on lack of speed or swiftness (skill), instead of focusing on best effort.

* Sticking to only one mode instead of utilizing several (e.g., always doing burpees HIIT rather than alternating on other HIIT days with, say, the switch jump and incline running on your treadmill).

* Performing HIIT less than 90 minutes after a full meal. Ideally, you should wait two hours after a full meal. However, a small snack shortly before the session, like a banana, is fine.

* Waiting longer than an hour to eat after the session. HIIT at home means you can eat literally right after the session. Have something prepared and ready to enjoy right when the session is over. This is important because not only is your body

begging for recovery fuel (it gets a lot of it from stored fat, but it also relies on food), but right after HIIT, your glucose metabolism is in top gear.

* Ignoring an injury; attempting to work through it. If you notice pain or discomfort in your feet, knees or hips, cease the activity and take measures to heal the injury before resuming HIIT.

* Improper footwear

Chapter 16: Hiit Workouts For Beginners

HIIT workouts can be created depending on the fitness level of the individual. Even though this is a high stress routine, it is not restricted to advanced athletes alone. With a more relaxed pace and less stressful exercises, even beginners can get into HIIT workouts.

Before you start performing any HIIT exercises, remember that you cannot make this a part of your everyday routine. At most, HIIT can be performed twice a week, especially by beginners. This is because HIIT is an extremely stressful routine that really taxes the body. The body needs time to recover adequately after each HIIT session.

HIIT Beginner's Workout – 1

Duration - 21 minutes

This workout is designed to be performed on a treadmill. However, you can also perform it on an elliptical machine.

5 minutes – Warm up adequately before beginning this exercise. Keep the pace relaxed but exercise each muscle carefully.

3 minutes – Rest Interval – For 3 minutes, increase your speed and increase the incline on the treadmill by 1 %. This is your baseline now.

1 minute – Work Interval – Increase the incline further by 1% to 3% depending on your ability for 1 minute. Increasing the incline automatically increases the intensity of the workout.

3 minutes – Rest Interval – Decrease both the speed and the incline to bring yourself back to the baseline level.

1 minute – Work Interval – Increase your incline and speed again to attain the intensity of the previous work interval.

3 minutes – Rest Interval – Once again, come back to the baseline level to bring your heart rate to a comfortable level.

5 minutes – Cool Down – Decrease the incline and the speed further till you come back to a comfortable level before stopping the exercise completely.

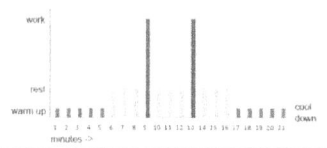

HIIT Beginner's Workout – 2

This is a slightly longer routine with a more complicated routine. It mixes jogging, sprinting and walking to create more levels of intensity.

Start your workout with a warm up session lasting 5 minutes, with stretches to prepare your muscles for the intense workout that follows.

Low Intensity – Brisk walk for 5 minutes without any incline on the treadmill.

Medium Intensity – Increase the intensity between 2% and 3% and continue walking briskly for 2 minutes.

High Intensity – Once again, remove the incline and run or sprint for 1 minute at maximum intensity.

Medium Intensity – Jog without any incline for 2 minutes to reduce the intensity slightly.

High Intensity – Jog at an incline of 2% to 4% for 1 minute.

Low Intensity – Remove the incline again and walk briskly for 5 minutes.

Medium Intensity – Increase the incline once more to 2% to 3% and walk briskly for 2 minutes.

High Intensity – Remove the incline and run or sprint on the treadmill for 1 minute.

Medium Intensity – Remove the intensity and jog for 2 minutes.

High Intensity – Jog for 1 minute at an incline of 2% to 4%.

Low Intensity – Walk briskly without an incline to lower the intensity for 3 minutes.

The entire workout lasts 35-40 minutes and can be done on a treadmill.

Finish the workout with a cool down session for 5 to 10 minutes. Include stretches in the cool down to relax your muscles after the exercise.

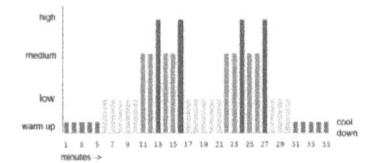

HIIT Beginner's Workout – 3

This is a swimming workout targeted at those who prefer the pool to a gym. Before you engage in a pool workout, ensure that you have perfected the method of swimming. If you do not use the appropriate techniques, you might end up damaging your muscles in a high intensity workout.

Start with a warm up session of 10 minutes. Warming up is essential for all exercises and especially for HIIT exercises. In an Olympic sized pool, swim two to three laps to warm up your system appropriately.

High Intensity – For 45 seconds, sprint at a high velocity in freestyle. Push yourself as far as you can go to achieve maximum intensity.

Medium Intensity – Paddle or swim lightly for 90 seconds to recover your breath and your system' functions.

Continue alternating between the two intensities for 15 minutes to complete the HIIT part of your workout.

When you are done, cool down for at least 10 minutes by swimming laps at a normal pace or by hitting the treadmill and walking at a low intensity.

Tips and Warnings

-       If you prefer to focus on weightlifting to remain fit, you can easily incorporate HIIT into your workout. Weightlifting is, by itself, an interval workout. As a result, all you need to do is up the intensity. You can increase the intensity by increasing the load you lift.

-       Changing up exercises keeps the body from adjusting to one particular workout. Thus, experiment with different kinds of exercise, such as running, swimming, jumping, skipping and so on.

You can also switch exercises within the same routine. If you start with running, make the next set a skipping set. This keeps your body on its toes and provides you with much better results. As a side benefit, you also will keep your interest alive and boredom away.

- Beginners should take care that they do not overstrain their muscles. While HIIT does provide many benefits, it requires a fit body to perform these workouts. Do not immediately start at a high intensity. Work up to the required intensity over a few weeks. Give your body approximately two weeks to adjust to each new intensity before you decide to increase it. Otherwise, you run the risk of causing serious injury to various parts of your body that are not yet ready to handle high intensity and strain.

-      If you find your motivation flagging after a certain period of time, it helps to remind yourself of your objectives. If you wish to lose a certain amount of weight, imagine how you would look after you achieve your goal, or write down your goal to help keep your motivation up.

HIIT workouts for beginners are specifically designed to help them improve their shape so that they can handle high intensity workouts after a while. Beginners should ensure that their stance and techniques are proper before embarking on HIIT workouts to reduce the amount of possible damage.

As one's stamina and capacity increases, one can move on to intermediate workouts that require more resources and demand an increased level of fitness.

Chapter 17: Sample Hiit Workouts For Intermediate

* Rotation jump. This will be challenging; do 15 second bursts with 1-2 minutes of recovery.

* Quartet x 2: Mountain climber, floor bunny hop, jog in place, jumping jacks. Eight cycles total, but each exercise here represents the first four cycles. Repeat them again for the second four cycles. Take 90 seconds to two minutes in between for recovery.

* Staircase top lunge. Use the floor with the first stair. Eight cycles with two minute rests. The top lunge is also called a reverse lunge.

* Tuck jump. Do this before a mirror if possible. The difference between intermediates and advanced here is speed and knee height. Six cycles, one minute rest intervals.

* Jump rope. If you can continue jumping after 30 seconds, jump faster and/or higher. This will be taxing to attempt, but an all-out effort for even 15 seconds is HIIT. Aim for a 15 second blast for eight sets; apply Fartlek rests.

Sample HIIT Workouts for Advanced

* Squat jump. Focus more on jump height before squat depth so that a burn in the quadriceps doesn't force you to stop prematurely. Eight cycles, 1-2 minute rest. For a madder routine, do this Tabata style. (Note the modification differences in the trainees.)

* Box jump Tabata. Use at least an 18 inch height: 20/10, 20/10, etc.

* Lunge jump/lateral jump. If you have "bad knees," don't do this. Complete a scissor jump (aka lunge jump) on both sides, then leap both feet together and move right into a jump to one side, then the other, then return both feet together; from there go back into the scissor jumping. Eight cycles, 1-2 minute rest.

* Staircase dash (one or two steps at a time). Do Tabata. This will scorch. Enough stairs are required so that you can cover a continual ascent for 20 seconds: multiple flights in your apartment building or outside your condo.

* Staircase bunny hop/back hop. Rather than a nonstop ascent, use one flight of stairs, because when you get to the top (which may take less than 10 seconds, but

don't go longer than about 15 seconds with the continual ascent), you will then bunny hop back down—backwards.

Warning: This requires athleticism. Practice in slow motion first to make sure you're not at risk for stumbling or falling backwards. Lean forward to prevent falling backwards.

The work interval consists of hopping up and down in this fashion until 30 seconds are up, but make sure your modification makes more than 30 seconds impossible. Besides speed, manipulate intensity with height of the backwards/downward jump, and/or adding a squat to it!

HIIT Progression

* One key to progression is to be consistent. Skipping workouts will prevent progression or greatly slow it down. Commit to two to three times a week, and

make the HIIT days the same each week, though this isn't necessary, but it will help you keep more committed.

* Another way to avoid skipping sessions is to never, never believe you can replace a session with an unusually rigorous bout of housework or yard work. No matter how "bushed" cleaning the attic, raking the leaves, shovelling the snow or helping a friend move made you feel, if these tasks occurred on a HIIT day, your HIIT slot still remains open! You must still do your HIIT.

* When you track progression, you're motivated to get better and better. When possible, keep track of number of jumps, depth, height, how you feel (RPE), etc. You will know when you're progressing. If you're using cardio equipment, keeping track is easy by noting speeds, inclines and RPMs. Another feature of progression is

having to use light hand weights to reach the same RPE.

* Progression can be aided with apps that have progression-tracking features.

* Strength train. Working out with weights will strengthen your joints and improve overall fitness, which will help reduce joint strain during HIIT.

Chapter 18: Visualization Techniques

Now that you really know about the secrets & laws of attraction through the use of Visualization procedures, you really need to keep in mind that you need to fix your mind first, before you can easily use your power of imagination to attract success to yourself. Mind-fixing should be just gradual because it helps you eliminating the past negative thoughts while you simply focus on more positive thoughts.

Before you believe in your goal, you really need to have an idea of what exactly it looks like. You need to see it before you believe it. Visualization helps you simply create a mental image of future events you want in your entire life, when you simply visualize a desired outcome, you've a glimpse of its eventuality, & are motivated to pursue the goal. Through visualization you can easily create your desired future. Visualization shouldn't be seen as a gimmick rather it's such a well-developed method for improving your performance towards achieving your goals & desires.

Visualization Techniques steps

Imagination- Draw a realistic plan for yourself & break them into smaller units that're achievable. Give yourself sufficient time-frame to achieve each stage in a way that you really do not place too much pressure on yourself.

Coordination- Coordination is such a visualization technique that actually helps you reduce your fear & anxiety about achieving your future. The purpose of using coordination in Visualization is to achieve your goals by using the one-step-at-a-time approach. You really do not have to rush through as most people want to, rather, take a simple & gradual approach.

Concentration- this steps simply allows you to follow your dreams with poise, & perfection, without losing focus. Athletes for instance can easily make use of visualization techniques to increase their performances by focusing at breaking one record at a time- they really tend to break their own records before attempting to break world records.

There're basically 2 types of visualization;

-Outcome visualization- this entails the envisioning of your goal, trough the creation of a mental image alongside the desired outcome just by using all your senses. Make sure you hold on your mental image as close as possible, & when you imagine the satisfaction & excitement of making it to the finish line, you'll be motivated to the end.

- Process Visualization is such a type of visualization that actually allows you envision each of the necessary actions you must just take to achieve the final results you want.

Chapter 19: The Essentials Of Hiit

HIIT Training can give some amazing results if performed correctly. However, there are a few essentials that you need to consider before starting HIIT. For instance, features like the duration of this routine, the equipment you require and the extent to which you need to go in terms of intensity of the workout are important.

What Equipment To Use In HIIT?

Beginner HIIT training can be fairly effective with just your body weight, but as you move along, you may want to introduce some equipment into your routines.

HIIT training can be done using an assortment of methods. You can work with anything from a Stairmaster to a bike or treadmill and even incorporate sprinting, bicycle sprints or elliptical workouts.

But whichever machine or activity you choose, you need to do it hard, fast and only stop when you feel that you can't possibly push any further.

A popular choice for HIIT in this regard is a treadmill. It is best to use a curved treadmill since this provides a full body workout. Another common choice for high intensity workouts is the stationary bike to accelerate heart rate and keep it pounding there.

An arm bike is also a good machine to use during high intensity workouts. Working out on this machine requires maximum effort and wrestlers have been using it for building their strength for a long time.

However, if you do not have the budget for all these machines or a gym membership, you can simply get a jump rope. A jump rope will get your heart rate up and keep it there for the duration of the workout.

If you want to follow a somewhat no-equipment HIIT plan, then stick with moves like jumping jacks, sprinting or sprinting in place, and high knees to get your heart going.

How Intense Should The Workouts Be?

High intensity workouts are cardio workouts that are aimed at getting the maximum effort in a short period of time. The key is to keep the intensity levels at the maximum.

But for the workout to be effective, you need to determine your own intensity level. For a beginner, the intensity of a HIIT routine will be different from someone who has been doing it for a while. The sets are short in duration, ranging from 20 to 90 seconds but they require full body force. If you feel that you can continue a routine for more than 30 minutes, then chances are that you are not working at maximum intensity.

HIIT is more popular as compared to other methods because it burns calories more rapidly. It has been seen through research that the more intense a workout is, more fat is burnt. Normally, fitness experts judge the intensity level suitable for a person using the RPE scale or the rate of perceived exertion scale.

This scale basically has a 1-10 spectrum, with 10 being the point where you give the workout everything you have got. Every person needs to determine where they stand on this spectrum and try to move to

10 by gradually upping the intensity of their workouts.

Conclusion

It is with hope that your HIIT related questions have been answered. May this book help you achieve your workout goals, whether it's to lose weight, build strength, or to increase your stamina. May this book encourage and challenge you to try basic HIIT programs. It doesn't matter if you start with light routines as long as you gradually increase and change your exercise programs. HIIT works best when you can feel muscle pain, but don't overtrain.

For best results as you undergo HIIT, it's advisable to make healthy eating choices. The best thing about HIIT is there are no food restrictions and scheduled eating plans. However, do not over-indulge in junk food and sugary foods because it will make you feel sluggish and decrease your overall health. After all, do you want your effort of undergoing HIIT to be put to waste? I don't think so.

So the next time you want to eat, take a small portion, but do not over-indulge. Remember, 1 slice of pizza takes 70 minutes of running to burn.

Reread the guidelines on how to get started on HIIT; if you're not feeling any body pain after your training then you're not exerting enough effort. Don't be discouraged and try again. Challenge yourself to an exercise routine that would require you to give 100% effort. Remember the term, "No Pain, No Gain". Literally, if you don't feel any pain, there'll be no muscle gain.

www.ingramcontent.com/pod-product-compliance
Lightning Source LLC
Chambersburg PA
CBHW060322030426
42336CB00011B/1164